ACKNOWLEDGMENTS

Big thanks to Kenneth A. Wightman, MS, ND; JMK, and Gayle K.

I0441004

FORWARD

Voice Tells No Lies is about how the resonance of voice is used in a technology called EVox to access quantum fields. Our clients use the EVox technique to cope with the emotional aspects of stress and most recently to drive out mycoplasma like organism that seem to 'lock' up energetic fields. There are a number of conspiracy theories about government 'weaponize' mycoplasma. We are only concerned that a number of our clients present with mycoplasma and have found no other ways to clear it. Once mycoplasma has been confirmed after being indicated by the Zyto instrument, the EVox is used to drive the organism out energetically. A handset facilitates an electronic bio-communication between the subject and the Zyto instrument. This handset can be mailed to an individual and the scan performed remotely from the clinician. The digital electronic communication is a beneficial electromagnetic field (EMF) signal. The EMF signal counters negative (unhealthy) tones recorded in the subject's voice to reframe perspectives in 12 different emotional zones. When a subject discusses each member of their family the technique is called Transgenerational Reframing (TGR). TGR takes into accounts perspective over several generations. The Case Studies included illustrate the spectrum issues that clients use the EVox for and the variety their feedback.

This manual is to help answer the question, "How does it work?" This is difficult to explain because scientists do not yet completely understand how quantum physics works. Some clients don't care how it works they just care if it will work for them! Let me ask, "Do you have to understand everything about the voltage, resistance and amperage of electricity before you switch the light on?" It is nice if you know the physics but it is not necessary to take advantage of being able to illuminate the room. The same is true with EVOX. It is fun to discuss what we know and what we theorize but don't let this get in the way of getting beneficial results. Like the first lay person that switched on a light, it is important to know that EVOX is not going to electrocute or harm you in anyway. Also, know that the results are illuminating even if you, "Don't get it."

INTRODUCTION

We have several different examples of cymatics, the science of how sound affects materials, that can be viewed on line. Dr. Emoto's experiments show how water restructures according to specific words. We can see how different vibrations can determine different shapes in the sand. There is evidence in cydonian architecture that giant stones may have been levitated into place and perhaps even reshaped by sound. In South Africa we can see from the sky what looks likes microchips and amplifiers made from stones. Experts think that sound was used in these structures to mine precious metals from the earth. There is an example in the Bible that used sound to demolish three feet thick fortress walls that surrounded an entire city.

Under close micro-examination of our body's cells we can see structures that look like capacitors, transistors and microchips. The ancient Egyptians believe that our pineal gland is a receiver and our pituitary gland is a transmitter. Receiving and transmitting to what and for what purpose?

The science of quantum physics helps us to understand soundwave like particles make up the most fundamental units of all matter in existence. That some subatomic particles are virtual in that they are in this dimension of existence for a period of time and then in another dimension another period of time. In other words, sometimes they are there and sometimes they are not. Everything in our universe is part of and is comprised of the quantum field. All matter in the universe is interconnected by quantum waves which have no boundary. Matter itself is made of waves. Matter can be purposed into physical reality from the wave nature of the quantum field. Quantum field is a subset of the zero point field. The quantum field occurs as a result of the interaction of the electromagnetic waves of the zero point field and the subatomic particles of the quantum field. The interaction results in scalar waves. Scalar Waves do not have direction or spin but in reality are interference patterns that are transformed via a holographic fournier transformation into material reality. This transformation is conducted by consciousness.

You just read that matter can be purposed into reality, thoughts can be transformed into matter by our consciousness and our pineal gland is a receiver and our pituitary gland is a transmitter. Many questions still remain, "How, why and for what purpose?" Some describe an ordered quantum field that surrounds us. It is thought that what keeps us from tapping into this ordered quantum field is doubt, insecurity, confusion, distraction, fear, anger, disconnect, false beliefs, critical/negative thinking, unforgiveness, and distrust. These low resonating frequency emotions are like static in our source connection. Perhaps ancient man was more sophisticated, more in tune with telepathic and telekinetic abilities. There are recent reports that scientist have achieved laser beam using teleportation.[1]

The ordered quantum field represents resonance of balance and health and disorder is represented by destructive resonances. The EVOX seems to neutralize these frequencies of disorder and improve our reception which changes our perception. The sessions are stronger when a Zyto scan is in combination with EVox because there are always more things going on than what we know or think. The combination is a better balanced or holistic approach to the total person.

I do not know where the "Ordered Quantum Field" is or how it is accessed by any other method but I am confident it is created, and controlled by God.

Table of Contents

---

[1] https://phys.org/news/2016-03-star-trek-vision-reality.html

I. How EVOX works

A. Procedure

Step 1

Decide what topic is to be discussed

Step 2
Place headset over ears and microphone near mouth.

Step 3
Speak into the microphone until the voice map generated by the software is complete.

Step 4
Continue the action of step 3 until a Releasing Pattern or Dynamic Shift is indicated.

B. Behind the scenes

The handset facilitates an electronic bio-communication between the subject and the Zyto instrument[2]. The digital signal pings the subject's hand electrical meridian end points in response to the voice tones. This electronic communication is a beneficial electromagnetic field (EMF) signal with a binary code of "yes" or "no". The EMF signal received by the subject neutralizes specific negative (unhealthy) frequencies. The goal of each session is a Releasing Pattern. Releasing Patterns are indicated by the computer program and requires three consecutive decreases in voice tone emotional intensity. Follow up includes indicating subtle perception changes experienced by the subject.

C. Session Options

1. Single session EVOX: for Individual Specific Perspectives. EVOX technique records the voice and indicates intensity of the emotional zones by the recorded tones present in the voice and adds back the ones that are missing. Ideal for: Phobias, Addictions, Eating Disorders, PTSD, Abuse, Severe Trauma, Injury, Learning Disabilities, Foggy Thinking, Relationships, Performance Writer's block, Disabling Inhibitions, Stuck in a rut, Goal setting, and Confidence at work.

2. Multiple Session Transgenerational Reframing (TGR): for Global Perspectives where genetic inertia is holding one in a static pattern (see Glossary). TGR breaks the genetic inertia that holds one in a static rut. Ideal for issues of : Health, Wealth, Happiness, Love of Life, Success in Business, Love of Self, Acceptance of Change, Accountability, Self Expression, Peace, Open to Possibilities, Self Validation, Self Accepting, Human Potential, Enlightenment, and Compassion. Transgenerational Reframing (TGR) series is generally conducted in a minimum of 5

---

[2] http://www.zyto.com/EVOX.html

sessions to address: Architectural design of relationships, Voice Map Recording for each family member, Transitional Shifts for 1-8 members per session and Post Self recording

D. Optimizing Sessions

1. Releasing patterns occur sooner if the subjects can address the heart, root or core of the issue from the beginning of the session. When they are able to visualize the person, place or event that stirs the most intense emotion, the specifics words they choose are not important. The subject may choose to discuss specifics by choosing words that help trigger their emotional memory. They continue to focus their attention on the core issue through the session. I am available during the session to guide and assist. There are times when I have helped them formulate phrases, affirmations or I AM statements to nail an intention. Many times during a session, I have observed a sweet spot when the subject experiences a revelation, a self discovery or awareness. I call this sweet spot event, breaching the hull or reaching the core of the issue. Sometimes they begin to answer their own questions or creative juices begin to flow that help them with resolutions. Almost always following this experience, a releasing pattern is displayed.

2. The Zyto is equipped to make homeopathic remedies. This is achieved by capturing the electronic digital imprint in water. We call it energized water. The subject drinks half after the session and the rest before they go to bed. The goal is to reinforce the energy imprint or vibrational frequency of the Releasing Pattern within the same circadian rhythm in which it was achieved. Affirmation statements accomplish this same purpose.

3. Our program, *Significance Journey* based on *The Search For Significance* book by Robert McGee, may be recommended before or after a session. It is our way of helping people identify core issues. This is discussed further in section III. A. Education on page 8.

E. Technology Background

1. EVOX: E in EVox is for Emotion.

2. VOX: the Latin word for voice. EVOX alters cellular memory using a biofeedback technology. Events are interpreted, transcribed into an electrical signal, and stored with an emotional tag. Connective tissue storage is a matrix language of vibration frequencies[3]. Vibration

---

[3] Pim van Lommel writes in his book "Consciousness Beyond Life" (2010)

language can be recorded, erased (cleared), tuned, stored, or altered. Cells echo stored frequencies and reinforce perspectives[4]. EVOX monitors 12 Zones of perspectives that influence our emotions and frame the view of our reality. Voice carries a clue of what emotional energy is stored in tissue. Lie detectors monitor stress in the voice and the body as one is responding to questions. This is just the tip of the iceberg! The voice cannot produce what the ear does not hear[5]. The converse is that your voice produces what people have told you about yourself and what you have believed to be true. Voice mapping based on Tomatis Voice Theory[6].

3. Technique developed from the following predecessors

A. Galvanic skin response (GSR[7]) skin conductance can be used as a measure of emotional and sympathetic responses[8].

B. Skin Conductance Response (SCR) is highly sensitive to emotions in some people. Fear, anger, startle response, orienting response, and sexual feelings are all among the reactions which may produce similar skin conductance responses. These responses are utilized as part of the polygraph[9] or lie detector[10]. Individuals can use these technologies to foster positive emotions and psychophysiological coherence. They can effectively initiate a repatterning process, whereby habitual emotional patterns underlying stress are replaced with new, healthier patterns that establish increased emotional stability, mental acuity, and physiological efficiency as a new familiar baseline or norm.

C. A needleless technique called ElectroAcupuncture (EAV) was developed by Voll. His publications discuss *Emotional Stress, Positive Emotions, and Psychophysiological Coherence*[11].

4. *Lie To Me* is a TV series which focuses on emotional facial micro gestures. Recently an episode featured an instrument that

---

[4] Candace Pert, author of Molecules of Emotion

[5] http://en.wikipedia.org/wiki/Alfred

[6] http://en.wikipedia.org/wiki/Alfred

[7] http://en.wikipedia.org/wiki/Skin_conductance

[8] *Physiology of Behavior.* New Jersey: Pearson Education, Inc. ISBN 978-0-205-23939-9.

[9] http://en.wikipedia.org/wiki/Polygraph

[10] http://en.wikipedia.org/wiki/Lie_detector

[11] IHM researchers McCraty and Dana Tomasino chapter in 2006 book, *Stress in Health and Disease*, published by Wiley-VCH.

measures voice stress that the ear cannot hear. The series interest is people lying to each other. We want to help people to stop lying to themselves.

II. Clinical Practice Application

Many people come to our clinic because they feel really bad and want us to help. For some, even though all of their physical parameters are resolved, they still don't achieve their optimal level of wellness. It is as if they subconsciously reject becoming physically well, undeserving of being well or guilty if they became well. We started using the Zyto EVOX to find out if some physical issues have emotional connections and if voice mapping is an effective resolution. We are thrilled when a client feels empowered to say something like, "This is the emotional root of my cancer, my breakdown or fatigue." Addressing emotional roots that manifest physically is our focus for using the EVOX.

A. Conventional treatments for emotional problems are not enough

Dismal stress and depression statistics emphasize a growing problem in the American population. This problem is exacerbated by not enough successful treatments or approaches for addressing life's stressors that cause severe unhappiness. The following are some of the stress, unhappiness and depression statistics:

- According to the 2008 Harris Poll[12] only 1 out of 3 Americans is happy
- Use of antidepressant pharmaceuticals has risen 400%[13] since the 1990s
- The top selling pharmaceutical of 2013 was Abilify[14]
- The 2004 CDC statistics available show that suicide is on the rise[15]
- 75 to 90% of all visits to primary care physicians results from stress-related disorders 1991[16]
- Depression is the most common type of mental illness, affecting more than 26% of the U.S. adult population and expected to

---

[12] http://www.huffingtonpost.com/2013/06/01/happiness-index-only-1-in_n_3354524.html?

[13] http://www.webmd.com/depression/news/20111019/use-of-antidepressants-on-the-rise-in-the-us

[14] http://www.drugs.com/stats/top100/sales

[15] http://www.sciencedaily.com/releases/2007/09/070907221530.htm

[16] Paul Rosch, MD., President , American Institute of Stress http://www.stress.org/americas-1-health-problem/

become the second leading cause of disability throughout the world, trailing only ischemic heart disease[17]
- Major depression will be the 2nd cause of death in the world by 2020[18]
- Cultural hopelessness, or when people think that "this is all there is," is linked to depression[19]

The term "unhappiness" is used generally to express a perspective. It insinuates living a life less than fulfilling without resolution.

B. A new approach

Using depression as an example, our naturopathic protocol would address the condition as multifaceted. Depression is a "symptom" resulting from nutrient depletions, wounds, and imbalances of mind, body or spirit. The physical approach would be to balance the gut, metabolism, hormones, and neurotransmitters and look for emotional roots.
- "Gastrointestinal" Poor absorption can prevent the building block components from being available to maintain hormone and neurotransmitter balance.
- "Metabolism" Enzymes may not be available to convert building block components into the (hormone and neurotransmitter) metabolites - necessary to complete reactive pathways to their end point.
- "Hormones" like cortisol, DHEA, estrogen, progesterone, and testosterone have vital roles in stress, emotion, anxiety and reaction responses.
- "Neurotransmitters" like serotonin, dopamine, glutamate, epinephrine and norepinephrine play a similar role as hormones.

The supplement tools that are most commonly used to correct deficiencies and help support balance are: probiotics, enzymes, 5MTHF, B vitamins, trimethylglycine (TMG), S-adenosylmethionine (SAMe), tryptophan, 5-hydroxytryptophan (5HTP), gabapentin (GABA). Hormones can be addressed using bioidentical hormone replacement therapy (BHRT), but the first line of approach is to support the body in improving the metabolism of its own production. Herbs that support endocrine function contain phytosterols such as Black Cohosh, Chaste Tree, Swiss Green Oat, Tribulus, Rehmania, and Andrographis. Herbs that support neurotransmitter function include St. John's Wort and Valerian Root. It is

_____

[17] http://www.cdc.gov/mentalhealth/basics.htm

[18] David Scheiderer, MD, Psychoneuroimmunologist

[19] http://www.sheldrake.org/books-by-rupert-sheldrake

recommended that the effectiveness of these supplements be tracked with analytic testing.

If the subject does not respond to nutraceuticals, pharmaceutical or counseling, then EVOX is recommended. Some request EVOX before they begin any other approach.

III. Candidate Education and Paperwork

A. Education

We assist in determining those most likely to benefit from EVOX and how to optimize their session(s). As mentioned previously, we may recommend our *Significance Journey Program* if a subject indicates performance, approval, blame and shame as struggles or as behavior addictions. The TGR vs EVOX Determination Chart on page 18 correlates these behavior addictions with individual or genetic traumas. Please consider the following: If you wake up one morning with a hurting finger and realize you have a sliver that needs to be removed, your first instinct is not to track down where the sliver came from but to remove the sliver. Afterwards, it may be helpful to figure out where the sliver was picked up to that you do not do it again. Using this same reasoning, working on an issue is more important than figuring out where it came from. The programs and charts might help in understanding when problems started developing, how your family might have been the influencing factors and how behaviors become addictions. But understanding the problem doesn't do the work necessary to solving the problem.

The following are other aspects to consider in maximizing the EVOX experience:

1. Dispel fears of having to "spill their guts" to yet another person and going through the same old rigmarole.

- The candidate is not required to relay personal, private or confidential information. It is not "Talk Therapy".
- This is a new, non-invasive approach that specifically addresses the harmful results of negative emotion(s).
- The practitioner does not have to communicate with the exception of simple directions of "speak", "stop speaking" and "put your hand on the handset".
- The practitioner communicates with the candidate from their belief position when possible. (Please see Glossary for more

information on specific terminology. We are Christian and only bring beliefs into the conversation when asked.)
- The Emotional Self Assessment below may help people decide if they should call for an appointment:

Emotional Self Assessment

1. Y or N Is there any cause for concern about depression for you or your family?

2. Y or N Are there fears/phobias or anger issues that you have inherited from your parents or grandparents?

3. Y or N Do you believe that you will inherit a family member's physical or mental disease?

4. Y or N When you talk about yourself, do you use words that tell others you are not happy and healthy?

5. Y or N Does your appearance tell others that you are not happy and healthy?

6. Y or N Do the items in your grocery cart or on your restaurant receipt tell others that you are not happy and healthy?

7. Y or N Were you raised with more criticism than affirmation?

8. Y or N Are you fearful, angry or worried more times than not?

9. Y or N Are your emotions controlling you more than you are in control of your emotions?

10. Y or N If you met yourself at a party, would you think you were good company?

11. Y or N Are you exhausted with disappointed in others or disappointed in yourself?

12. Y or N Have people said that you talk angrily, too loud, too soft or have an unhealthy tone in your voice?

13. Y or N Are you overwhelmed, overly-stressed or beyond unhappy?

14. Y or N Have you ever shared a deep issue with a therapist or friend and felt un-helped or even worse afterwards?

15. Y or N Do you shove feelings down deeper and deeper out of self preservation?

16. Y or N Have you given up on feeling better and just struggle to get through each day?

17. Y or N Are you looking for something different to help you emotionally?

18. Y or N Do you have unexplained fears, phobias or compulsions?

19. Y or N Have counseling and pharmaceuticals failed you for your emotional issue?

20. Y or N Are you interested in more information about our approach to emotional balance?

If your answered YES to 3 or more of the above questions, you are encouraged to contact Concepts In Wellness at 302-495-9620 or conceptsiw@gmail.com and make an appointment.

2. Explain the difference between good and bad electromagnetic field (EMF) energy

- EVOX is a form of good EMF. Bad EMF frequencies are from cell phones, Bluetooth, wireless, etc. These frequencies can be stored in biological systems in the form of electromagnetic oscillations[20]. A 2011 International Agency for Research on Cancer (IARC) meeting concluded that RF-EMF (cell phones, wireless, cordless, Bluetooth) is possibly carcinogenic to humans.[21] Dr. Blank at Columbia University published voluminous data to support the damaging effects of EMF on DNA.[22] Dr. Blank says, "Mother Nature hides her secrets well but she never lies".[23]
- The body needs good electromagnetic fields to function properly. Research has demonstrated that every cell in your body may have its own EMF. In his book *The Body Electric,* Robert Becker demonstrates that our cells actually communicate with each other via bioelectrical signals and electromagnetic fields. These natural EMFs help regulate important biochemical processes. Maintaining balance in those cellular electromagnetic fields is crucial to physical health.[24] EMF affects emotional disorders and mental conditions. When exposure to bad EMFs is reduced, healing energies flow more freely in the body. The nervous system and acupuncture meridian system are released from constriction and calmness sets in. The pineal gland increases its production of hormones and important chemicals that control and affect physical, emotional and mental functioning. There is also an increase in overall energy. Cells no longer function as though in a state of emergency.[25]
- Steve Sinatra's [MD Cardiologist] book, *Earthing* introduces the principle of "grounding" or our need to be connected to the earth's EMF. The earth's surface is negatively charged and contact with the earth allows electrons to neutralize free radicals in the human body. One study showed a reduction in blood viscosity and blood pressure, a key factor in cardiovascular disease. This can be accomplished by lying or walking barefoot on grass, sand or earth, or by lying on a special

---

[20] http://www.oscillatorium.com/id22.html

[21] http://www.arpansa.gov.au/radiationprotection/EMR/literature/june11.cfm

[22] Blank, PhD, College of Physicians and Surgeons, Columbia University. 2012. http://www.bioinitiative.org/report/wp-content/uploads/pdfs/sec07_2012_Evidence_for_Stress_Response_Cellular.pdf

[23] http://www.youtube.com/watch?v=Cx0VmLUDF48

[24] *The Body Electric,*' researcher and author Robert Becker

[25] http://www.earthcalm.ca/index_files/EMF_health_risks.htm#.Uupw-D1dXTo

pad connected to the earth by grounding wires or a rod, or plugged into a wall outlet with a "modern earth ground system[26]
- Our clinic provides guidance and resources[27] for people to protect themselves against harmful EMF. We provide some EMF guards that are disguised as bracelets or pendants. These products function under the premise that minerals or gems of the earth emit good EMF which neutralizes or deflects harmful EMF.

3. Types of people who have used EVOX: Administrator, Actors, Athlete, CEO, CFO, Child, Clerk, Director, Doctor, Electrician, Engineer, Father, Mother, Musician, Patient, Pilot, Public Speaker, Minister, Manager, Security Guard, Student, Teacher, Teenager, Wife, and Writer.

4. The technique may be helpful in individuals with stress, anxiety, obesity, depression, difficult relationships, losing loved ones, problems on the job and performance issues to name a few.

B. Intake forms

In the initial intake before beginning a session, the candidate's paperwork includes questions to assess the influences of the following:

1. Near Death Experiences, NDE: Those who have had NDE experiences may have altered EMF[28] and have a different reaction using the EVOX.

2. Outer Body Experiences, OBE: Those who have had OBE experiences may have an altered EMF and have a different reaction to using the EVOX.

3. Electrical Trauma and Exposure, ETE: Those who have had severe electrical shock, electrocution, or lightning strikes may have altered EMF and react differently to using the EVOX.

4. Electromagnetic Field, EMF Sensitivity[29]: Those who are sensitive to computers, watches, lights, and other common EMF[30] may react differently to using the EVOX.

---

[26] http://en.wikipedia.org/wiki/Stephen_Sinatra

[27] http://www.motherearthnews.com/natural-health/concerned-about-electromagnetic-fields-heres-what-you-can-do-to-minimize-risks.aspx#axzz34U7nPjKJ

[28] Journal of Transpersonal Research, 2012, Vol. 4 (2), 34-55

[29] http://www.emfanalysis.com/uploads/1/0/7/8/10781272/_wi-fi_7_legal_ramifications.pdf

[30] http://www.heartmath.org/free-services/articles-of-the-heart/energetic-heart-is-unfolding.html

5. Biometrics: Those with genetic or neurological predisposing indicators may react differently to using the EVOX.

6. Dreams[31]: If we consider that dreams relate emotion in symbols while asleep, then the EVOX may affect emotions in our unconscious dream state. We ask if there are any changes in dreams before or after each session.

7. Organ transplant recipients: Dr. Pearsall, MD discusses the transference of memories through organ transplantation[32]. We are interested to see if the transferred emotions[33] will respond to EVOX.

C. Schedule session(s)

Once the issues from the Topics Table on the next page have been reviewed, a determination of whether a single EVOX session or a five session Transgenerational Reframing (TGR) will be offered. After the session type is determined, core issues, intentions, and trigger words are noted.

---

[31] http://www.dreamcoach.com.au/

[32] http://www.paulpearsall.com/info/books.html

[33] Kate R uth Linton Knowing By Heart: Cellular Memory in Heart Transplants

IV. Emotions or Emotional Topics

Abandonment	Hard hearted	Pessimistic
Abused / Abuses	Hasty	Prideful
Addictions	Haughty	Procrastination
Always right	Heavy	Promiscuity (w/o love)
Anger	Hyper-achievement	Provoked
Anguish	Immature	Psychosis
Anxious	Impatient	Reflects on past failures
Attention Deficit	Incest	Rejected / Rejects
Avoidance	Indecisive	Repetitive Thinking
Betrayed / Betrayer	Independent	Reserved
Blamed/Blames	Inflexible	Rigid Beliefs
Broken	Inhibited	Second guessing
Burnout	Insecure	Self Critical / Critical
Circular Reasoning	Insensitive	Self Defeating
Condemnation	Insubordinate	Self Doubt
Conditional Love	Intimidated / Intimidating	Self Pity
Conflicting Beliefs	Intolerant / Intolerance	Self Sabotage
Confused	Invalidated	Selfishness
Contrite / Shame / Guilt	Irresponsible	Sensitive
Cruel	Irritable	Serious
Cult	Jealous	Sexual abuse
Defeatist	Joyless	Shut down
Defensive	Judgmental	Slob
Denial	Learning disabilities	Sorrowful
Depression	Legalistic	Stirred up
Disappointment/disappointed	Libido issues	Stressed
Disingenuous	Lies	Stubborn
Dissension	Life is too hard	Stuck
Doubt about creative art skills	Loss of Parent	Suppressed Emotion
Doubt about learning skills	Loss of Pet	Suppressed/Oppressive
Dream Terrors	Low esteem	Teased
Dread	Lukewarm	Timid
Emotionally disconnected	Manipulated/Manipulative	Trauma
Emotionless	Neglected / Neglectful	Troubled
Entertainer	Nightmares	Trust issues
Everything is a struggle	Non Compassionate	Unaccepting
False self confidence	Nonconfrontational	Acknowledgment
False self esteem	Oblivious	Unappreciated
Fatigue	Occupation Stress	Unaware
Fear	Office Politics	Undervalued
Fear of Confrontation	Opinionated	Undeserving
Fear of Failure	Out of Control	Unforgiven/unforgiveness
Fear of Loss	Overachiever	Unreasonable expectation
Fear of poverty	Overcompensating	Unwillingness
Fear of Rejection	Overindulge	Unworthy

V. Emotional Zones – Correlation of Negative to Positive

	Negative Zone Attributes	Positive Zone Attributes
1	**Acknowledgment**	**Self Validation**
	Stuck, Procrastination	Appreciation of individuality
2	**Repetitive Thinking**	**Creative Thinking**
	Defeated, Intimidated	Broaden perspectives
	Doubt about creative art skills	Effective problem solving
3	**Depression**	**Inner Peace**
	Reflects on past failures	Lives in the present
	Doubt about learning skills	Less worry & pressure
4	**Emotionally disconnected**	**Emotionally Integrated**
	Shut down	Connects easier with others
	Inhibited	Deeper Relationships
5	**Self Critical**	**Self Love**
	Hard hearted, Insensitive	Less blame & blaming
	Unaccepting, Non Compassionate	In touch with emotions
6	**Conditional Love**	**Unconditional Love**
	Always right, Manipulates	Maturity, Security
	Intolerant, Judgmental, Immature	Tolerance
7	**Anger**	**Acceptance of Change**
	Worry, Dread	Willingness
	Road rage	Openness, Flexibility
8	**Fear & Overwhelmed**	**Accountability**
	No fun	Balanced expectations
	Too serious	Courage
9	**Suppressed Expression**	**Appropriate Expression**
	Rejection	Compassion
	Nonconfrontational	Forgive offender
10	**Unworthy/Undeserving**	**Self Acceptance**
	Physical w/o love	Nurtured
	False self esteem, hyper achievement	Balance, Accepted
11	**Rigid Beliefs**	**Open Possibilities**
	Intolerance, Opinionated	Security
	Inflexible, Perfectionist	Less Doubt, Tolerance
12	**Conflicting Beliefs**	**Congruent Beliefs**
	Everything is a struggle	Connected, Effortless
	Life is too hard	Peace of mind

VI. Interpretation

A. Identify low frequency negative shifts to a perception vantage view

1. Voice is a spectrum of tone frequencies. The lower the frequencies, the more negative the correlating emotion. The emotional frequency is digitized to a binary code, presented to the body, and prioritized. The corresponding balancing frequency (raises or neutralizes the low frequencies) is transferred back to the body. When the low frequencies are removed it is like the dam breaks and creative energy can restore the

system.

2. Voice tones are like "tells" in a poker game
- Voice Tells that you can hear: Listen to someone's voice as they interview over the phone. You can sense a great deal from their voice such as, if they are standing up straight or slouching, if they are smiling or trembling. More importantly you can sense how much confidence they have - all because of their voice.
- Voice Tells that you may not hear: The 12 Emotional tones or zones that can be detected in your voice are - invalidated, defeated, depressed, disconnected, critical, unloved, anger, fear, rejected, unworthy, obstinate and confused.

3. After the EVOX bio-communication raises the subject's specific frequencies, look for the perception shift (See Emotional Zone Chart). Where a person felt defeated by a problem, now they can approach the problem from a new angle (Shift 2). Where a person was worrying or dreading a situation, now they are willing and open to talk to someone about the situation (Shift 7). Where a person was shut- down and cut-off, now they are willing to have a relationship and reconnect (Shift 4).

4. Connecting a shame issue to a spiritual issue: John Bradshaw in his chapter, "Healing the Shame that Binds You", refers to "toxic shame" as a rupture of the self with self, as an inner torment, a sickness of the soul, the hole in one's soul, sense of hopelessness, devastating soul murdering power, spiritual bankruptcy, and ultimately a spiritual problem. He says the "will" is disabled primarily to the shaming of the emotions. The shamed and blocked emotions stop the full integration of intellectual meaning. When an emotional event happens, emotions must be discharged in order for the intellect, reason, and judgment to make sense of it. Emotions bias thinking. As emotions get bound by shame their energy is frozen, which blocks the full interaction between the mind and will. He refers to the statement, "The greatest human power is the creative power."

I believe that EVOX documents the emotional energy discharge. It neutralizes or reduces the negativity from the individual's emotions, allowing creativity to mend the hole in the soul. Shame wounds the soul. Eve in the Garden of Eden believed a lie which was the first sin. The first negative emotion was shame. When we believe a lie about ourselves, we are vulnerable to shame.

B. Notice subtle changes

1. Volume and/or tone of voice change: Sometimes I hear the participant's voice tone change to strength and confidence. Individuals do not always express awareness of this voice volume or texture change.

2. Subject or context change: The subject matter might change to what resembles a resolution, conclusion or submission. I believe the conscience is dealing with each of the emotions that is presented and comes up with a plan, an approach and/or a perspective which is specific for the individual. Why the conscience doesn't do this anyway or all the time, how the EVOX exposes or deals with negative emotion, how perspective and intention changes behavior are still a mystery.

3. The fog lifts: I observe as the metaphorical "cloud" lifts, it seems as though the subject's consciousness begins to scan and look for core issues and resolutions. Now that the cloud is lifted, even a little, creativity can shine in. Where one was trapped, stuck, sinking, drowning, in a rut, shut down, stalled out and frozen - all of a sudden a window opens, answers come, engines start, a lifeline appears and a thaw begins.

4. Feeling lighter: People use terms like, "load", "burden" or "pressure" being lifted. It is as if we feel an actual physical weight pulling us down and shutting us down. The bible speaks of the spirit of heaviness. Several times I have noticed that when I am jogging, if I think of something negative, I stop jogging and begin to walk. I am not tired but weighed down. It is very typical that when someone finishes an EVOX session, they say that they feel lighter. They realize that the situation "doesn't go away", the offending person "doesn't change", and the lost "doesn't come back", but something changed within them.

5. Reaction or processing time changes: To be able to have more reaction time to think and process a response is a liberating and useful skill. The EVOX demonstrated improved responses in both adult and child subjects. The change in reaction time can be described using the analogy of a fuse. The length of the fuse determines how long it takes them to react to a situation. Typically when the fuse is very short, the reaction time is quick, the rational thinking time is non-existent and the situation does not turn out well. In my experience, EVOX helps lengthen the fuse. It helps subjects feel more in control and more confident. They are now more likely to stop taking abuse or causing abuse.

C. The power of perception

One of our clients wrote the following after several sessions: "We all know someone who really doesn't have better than average talent, but is very successful in life because he or she is so positive!" This person KNOWS he/she will be successful in work and relationships and has a confidence that draws people towards him/her in a productive, healthy way! Your perception is the reality that frames your life; forming boundaries within which you operate and trigger your behavior. Improve your perceptions and you will free yourself from negative ruts and enjoy life!

Imagine looking through a picture frame at a single quilt square. Until you back away and increase the field of view you will not see the blanket design. This is called reframing the perspective. Perception is the filter on the glasses through which you view the world and everyone in it. Perception is your reality and determines the outcome of your life. Reframe your emotional perceptions for a NEW REALITY!

The goal of the EVOX is to adjust the size of the frame or the filter of your conscious view or perception. When you can view a situation from a vantage point, you feel differently about the situation.

D. Generational Perceptions

Perception that is influenced from familial or close relationships requires the specific EVOX approach called Transgenerational Reframing (TGR).

- Scientific evidence indicates that certain memories are handed down through generations[34] as well as <u>fears and phobias</u>[35]. Researchers explain that extremely negative experiences can cause a chemical change on the DNA which is passed to future generations.

The study above supports a genetic and energetic link to emotions which TGR addresses. The idea that family relationship traits are passed from generation to generation has been observed by most of us. For example if your father was unloved and taught you to view life through the unloved filter, you assume people do not love you and it is difficult to love them; if the critical filter is over your eyes then you assume everyone is critical of you and you respond critically. Perhaps this has something to do with what is indicated in scripture. Exodus 34:7 says, "Yet he does not leave the guilty unpunished; he punishes the children and their children for the

---

[34] http://www.sciencegymnasium.com/2014/01/scientists-have-found-that-memories-may.html

[35] http://www.telegraph.co.uk/science/science-news/10486479/Phobias-may-be-memories-passed-down-in-genes-from-ancestors.html

sin of the fathers to the third and fourth generation." Perhaps the negative effects of sin are passed down like fears and phobias. The mechanics of how this happens biologically, genetically or spiritually are not known but on an energetic level, it seems to make more sense. The chart below suggests origins for the low frequency negative emotions.

TGR or EVOX Determination Chart

	Origin
	Origin
1	TGR: Trauma from misuse of reward & punishment method of raising children
	EVOX: Professional acknowledgement and belonging - Performance
2	TGR: Genetic doubts about creative arts & sports abilities
	EVOX: Skill competency - Performance
3	TGR: Genetic doubts about intellectual abilities
	EVOX: Haunted by past disappointments - Approval
4	TGR: Distracted parents
	EVOX: Fear of rejection and ridicule - Approval
5	TGR: Critical parents
	EVOX: Unforgiveness - Blame
6	TGR: Blames self for unkind, unloving, unresponsive behavior of caregivers
	EVOX: Passive aggressive - Blame
7	TGR: Family violence
	EVOX: Fear of loss & disappointment - Incomplete grieving - Shame
8	TGR: 1st or 2nd Born - Over responsible
	EVOX: Phobias - Shame
9	TGR: Affected by weakness, faults or abuse of parent or authoritative figure
	EVOX: Abandonment - Shame
10	TGR: Neglect, abuse or separation from mother
	EVOX: Confidence - Shame
11	TGR: Insecure from no positive father figure
	EVOX: Insecure - Shame
12	TGR: Trauma from generations
	EVOX: Overwhelmed - Shame

VII. Results

A. Case For Quantum Wellness

It wasn't until we had used the EVox for about two years that we learned an individual could verbally purpose, command, direct, and/or affirm themselves to heal from mycoplasmas using EVox. Once the Zyto indicates the mycoplasma resonance is present, the individual can EVox that specific organism. We have performed this protocol numerous times with successful results.

Weaponized Mycoplasma

There are allegedly, seven weaponized Mycoplasma variants that enter fluid and blood circulation that were created covertly by the U.S. government and are now wreaking havoc on the population are the following:
1.) M. Fermentans (incognitas strain). The term fermentans reveals fermentation process (i.e.: yeast, molds, fungus, spores, cancer).
2.) M. Penetrans penetrate the cell membrane and invade host cells.
3.) M. Pneumoniae attacks upper respiratory epithelial cells, inflaming them and causing upper respiratory infections and chronic pneumonia.
4.) M. Genitalium (Genitalia) invades urethral tissue and cells in the genital area causing pelvic inflammation and urethritis.
5.) M. Hominus is found in joint tissues in rheumatoid arthritis.
6.) M. Pirum is found in AIDS as a co-factor accelerating AIDS progression.
7.) M. Salivarium is found in salivary glands and joint tissues in rheumatoid arthritis.[36]

Mycoplasma fermentans (incognitus strain) probably comes from the nucleus of the *Brucella* bacterium. This pathogen was patented (US Patent No. 5,242,820, issued September 7, 1993) by the United States military and Dr Shyh-Ching Lo. Dr Lo is listed as the 'Inventor' and the American Registry of Pathology, Washington, DC, is listed as the 'Assignee' of 'Pathogenic Mycoplasma'. Dr Maurice Hilleman, chief virologist for the pharmaceutical company Merck Sharp & Dohme, stated that this disease agent is now carried by everybody in North America and possibly most people throughout the world.

Dr Charles Engel, who is with the US National Institutes of Health, Bethesda, Maryland, stated an NIH meeting on February 7, 2000: "I am now of the view that the probable cause of chronic fatigue syndrome and fibromyalgia is the mycoplasma..."[37]

Every organism in the universe possesses a **resonant frequency 'signature'**. Electro-medicine exposes a pathogenic organism to its resonant frequency and **causes it to self-destruct**.[38]

_____

[36] http://www.rense.com/general62/molecularterrorism.htm
[37] http://real-agenda.com/mycoplasma-the-linking-pathogen-in-neurosystemic-diseases/
[38] Dr. Leonard Horowitz http://educate-yourself.org/cn/naziflu28dec04.shtml

B. Case Studies

Case 1 (Myself)

I used EVOX to prepare for a difficult phone conversation. As anticipated, the person on the other end of the connection metaphorically dressed me down in a very personal way. Since my response was, "I'll get back to you," I feel this was a direct effect of EVOX because that is <u>not</u> how I normally react to insult. This result prompted me to confidently recommend EVOX to others.

Shift 2: Intimidation to creative solution.

After a client informed me that she was weepy for days after a unique session requiring 24 voice maps; I challenged myself to reproduce the same response. I completed my own TGR in two consecutive days with the same result (weepy). We now require a minimum of one day between each release or 10 voice maps.

In order to understand and optimize the technique; I've tried numerous methods looking to trip up the program. I have yet to do so. It is best not to overthink the process but let the energy do the work.

Case 2

A client doing a TGR spoke about her father in the following terms, "He is not my father, he was just a sperm donor, he hurt a daughter in every way a father could hurt a daughter." The EVOX session requires multiple voice recordings and she repeated the same sentence five times. The next session, she was very excited to report that she was telling her daughters about the EVOX session and told them she discussed her dad. She surprised herself in what she said. A session later remarked how good it is to say, "Her dad". She reported about a recent phone conversation, "Overall, I have more confidence. I just started saying "Wow" over and over because I realized I didn't have to tolerate what was being said to me. I stopped myself in mid-sentence and realize the animosity was gone!" This client had a noticeable improvement in the projection of her voice and confidence in her demeanor.

Shift 7: Family violence causing rage to willingness
Shift 9: Emotional abandonment causing passivity to self defense.

Case 3

A mother having trouble with her young adult son reports that in the heat of the battle, she did not engage. She said, "I am not going to take what he says personally". Also, this client had a family member that required several voice maps before a release occurred and found out by doing some family inquiry that there were many painful things that she did not know about this person.

Shift 3: Self doubt to less pressure
Shift 12: Generational trauma causing internal struggle to peace of mind

Case 4

A professional single woman suffering from the loss of her cat and being "unfriended" on Facebook in the same week. She reports that it helped with the losses and has helped her to be more patient. This client reported on several occasions that she could sense when the release was about to occur while she was speaking.

Shift 6: Judgmental to tolerant

Case 5

Five year old girl's parent reports that daughter is no longer hitting her sister in anger, is saying sorry after bursts of anger, not having meltdowns like before, and can laugh at herself. Whereas before, she was very sensitive about people who she perceived were laughing at her expense.

Shift 7: Threatened to flexible

Case 6

A woman overwhelmed by being an entrepreneur and mother of six children. She reported a new sense of acceptance for life which reduced her stress.

Shift 7: Worry to acceptance

Case 7

College student reported that his confidence was improved. He was attending a university where he knew no one and was far from home. After the session, he found it easy to make friends with fellow students during shared interests and activities.

Shift 4: Inhibited to connected

Case 8

Beaten by father, and traumatized by mother's neglect. "While on the phone I realized that there were two movies before me and I could play out either one. My typical response would have been rage, slam the phone down and cry or scream. Instead, I

wrapped the conversation up and said Goodbye." "When dealing with my two teenagers, I had emotional control and was assertive. They were shocked but responded with respect."
Shift 7: Rage to willingness

Case 9

Client was molested by a family friend while babysitting as a young teen. At the moment the EVOX indicated the release pattern, the electricity in the entire building suddenly went off. She became physically cold and weak and slumped back in her chair. She recovered in about 15 minutes.
Shift 6: Manipulated to maturity

Case 10

This client is a bedbound individual with severe rheumatoid arthritis. Her son had been kidnapped by an estranged ex husband and a virus took his life a few years after at the age of fourteen. She had been so frightened that he might be taken again that she kept him secluded and blamed herself for his death. After the EVOX session she said, "I realize that what I say to myself about myself because of the guilt, blame, and shame I feel about my son, is preventing my healing."
Shift 12: Confusion to clarity
Shift 5: Critical to self love

Case 11

Man who sacrifices for others at the expense of himself. He is a 24 hour caregiver for his wife and could only leave the home for not more than two hours at a time. He was a prisoner in his home. At the end of the session he was able to say, "I can better serve others if I take care of myself."
Shift 10: Undeserving to self acceptance

Case 12

Woman having marital issues; says her husband does not sleep with her, constantly brings up her weight gain and ruins every family meal by being critical. She says the EVOX has been primarily responsible for helping her to maintain emotional strength as she responds kindly to her husband; retraining him to be kind to her.
Shift 9: Rejection to compassion

C. Reported comments from Zyto Corp[39]

---

[39] Zyto Corp, Lindon, UT

1. Several subtle changes occurred within me during my first session, the power and impact of which became increasingly clear as time went on. The work and its impact deepened with the second session and I've been noticing positive differences in my moods, energy and attitude ever since.

2. I can't believe how much of life's junk does not bother me! This last session sort of knocked something loose. I'm doing so well, it is ridiculous!

3. Mean people & stressful situations have absolutely NO effect on me. I used to run from stressful situations and avoid possible conflict at all costs. I would literally start to have a panic attack. Gone! How cool is that! I keep thinking "I'm not freaking out about this or that."

4. I am so amazed and very pleased with the energetic shifts in my thinking, and noticeable changes in my behavior, which is the result of Perception Reframing sessions.

VIII. Conclusion

It was clear that subtle perception changes can cause dramatic changes in life experiences. I became curious about the impact that perception could have on consciousness and spirituality. How are mind, body and soul connected? How are we connected to other people and to God?

If our bodies are receptors of information, it is possible that our physical health conditions, diet defects, EMF exposure, or environmental influences can damage or interfere with these receptors. Unrealistic life expectations also interfere with maximizing our full potential. Often I hear subjects say, life wasn't supposed to be this way, so and so were not supposed to get a divorce, my daughter was not supposed to get pregnant, my father was not supposed to die. We are sad, upset, depressed, disappointed, frustrated, let-down, confused, or devastated because something didn't happen the way they were supposed to or someone didn't do what they were supposed to. When we have supposed expectations on life, we predestine our own judge and jury execution. In our mind, we agreed with a lie that we have control and then judged certain events and behaviors as a failure, deserving of fearful consequences. The cycle can be broken if we accept that it is okay if life doesn't turn out the way we thought it was supposed to.

I believe that EVOX helps remove, change or alter the destructive vibrational energetic frequencies that keep one from seeing a positive (true) reality. The result being; realization that the healing is already ours to enjoy!

It was God's word using his VOICE that created the universe. His voice energy is resonating in each of our atoms. Science has all but confirmed this by calling the smallest particles of the universe, quarks, as "God particles". They have sound wave characteristics and virtually appear and disappear into thin air.

We are created in His image. Our voice should reflect His image. 2 Timothy 1:7 says, "We are not given a spirit of fear, but of power and of love and of sound mind." The very voice of our creator is within us. Every atom of our existence resonates with the voice of our God and so should our voice!

The voice tells no lies.

IX. Additional Resources

These booklets are drawn from my practice experiences and for the education of my current, future clients and other interested parties. The other booklets besides *Voice Tells No Lies* are as follows:

Facing Stress: Learning stress prioritization can assist you in charting good and bad stress, understand the physical consequences of stress and develop a plan of action. I also discuss a supplementation protocol for thyroid, adrenal, hormones, sleep and inflammation based on customized testing and individual assessment.

Diex: Applying the Blood Type Diet and Spirit Temple Exercises to our daily routines reduces stress by fortifying our body (the transmitter, receiver and dwelling of the Holy Spirit). Learn stress relieving aspects of aromatherapy customized to blood type, earth elements and angelic symbolism. The 30 stress relieving Spirit Temple Exercise (Christian alternative to Yoga) positions are available at https://www.youtube.com/watch?v=u5lSxhzBQ0o.

Quantum Conscience: We can address the physical and spiritual aspects of consciousness, through 27 Equipping Visualizations, 12 Step Stress-aholic Meditations and dream journaling. This text is an excellent continuation of *Voice Tells No Lies* to exploring invisible aspects of bio-communication sessions. This information was compiled for clients expressing interest in spiritual terms and consciousness practices. It is presented without condemnation or religious induction but for the *"soul"* purpose of informing and educating.

Toxic-Free Gardening: Discusses the damaging effects of genetically modified organisms (GMO) and endocrine disruptors (EDS) in our food and environment.

Tracy's Inferno: Introduces each circle of my life crises as layers of comedy. "What is to give light must endure burning"--Victor Frankl

September Mourning: Science fiction historical mystery eschatological adventure novel.

A Disclaimer: None of the statements have been evaluated by the FDA. Furthermore, none of the statements should be construed as dispensing medical advice, making claims regarding the cure of diseases. You should consult a licensed healthcare professional before starting any therapy, supplement, dietary, or exercise program, especially if you are pregnant or have any pre-existing injuries or medical conditions.

Tracy Wightman, CCN, is a practitioner at Concepts in Wellness, conceptsiw@gmail.com, 302-495-9620, myconceptsinwellness.com, Concepts in Quantum Wellness: http://wp.me/P8EaHt-6 #ConceptsTLC and Significant Recovery Blog: conceptsinwellness.wordpress.com.

X. Glossary Introduction

I have tried to overcome communication hurdles or gaps between the Christian, Metaphysical, Science, and New Age Communities. For example, the bible may say Jesus "knew their thoughts" and other terms might be "read their minds, telepathy or remote viewing depending on how far away He was from them."

We have no excuse to pass judgments [most of us are hypocrites that do it anyway] Romans 2:1. Stop passing judgments [and instead try to figure out how to do the opposite] Romans 14:1.

To not use a method just because an opposing group uses it is like saying we cannot pray because people who believe differently pray.

GLOSSARY OF TERMS

A

Akashi Record: (Divine Word*) All knowledge exists somewhere out there. *See Information Field.*

Angels: Heavenly Spirit Guides or Godly Messengers

Anger: A low resonating frequency emotion that is stored as a cellular memory pattern and can contribute to poor clinical outcomes.

Armor or spiritual suit: Force Field or Energy Field

Atonement Healing Perspective: Recompense

Awakening: Awareness that brings revelation or a revelation that expands awareness.

B

Bach Remedies: High energy flower essence categorized by personality types and used to influence behavior.

Biometrics: In-utero neurological development indicators such as fingerprints, genetic predisposition of physiology or behavior such as blood type or lifestyle indicators such as earlobe creases.

Bosons: Bosons are particles with integer spin ($s = 0, 1, 2, ...$). They can either be elementary (like photons) or composite (such as mesons, nuclei or even atoms). There are five known elementary bosons: the four force carrying gauge bosons γ (photon), g (gluon), Z (Z boson) and W (W boson), as well as the Higgs boson.

C

Chakra: (Eye Singularity Perspective*) Energy points at the plexuses of veins, arteries and nerves.

Cellular Matrix Memory: The body never forgets an assault and our emotional field never forgets an insult. These traumas are recorded in connective tissue memory patterns

Clearing: bio-communication technology to erase vibration residual left behind from past physical and emotional traumas from the cellular matrix memory

Co-creator: Our participation in creation through our creativity.

Co-infector: Typically there are primary and secondary infectors in an infections. The secondary infectors are also called co-infectors.

Connective tissue matrix language: Vibration frequency signatures in tissues of our body.

Conscience: Our inner self and moral sense

Conscious: Aware state of consciousness

Consciousness: Aware of self existence and self awareness

Cymatics: (Jericho's Wall Collapsing Perspective*) (Joshua 6:20)
The science of sound as a tool. Sound waves used to shatter kidney stone (sonic), explode rocks, levitate objects, mine minerals out of the earth and break down the walls of Jericho.

D

Dream: An unconscious expression of emotion using symbols while we are asleep.
Dream Decoding: Interpreting emotional symbols; Dream Symbolism
1. Flying: Responsibility freedom; 2. Naked: exposed, defenseless; 3. Snakes: change, manipulation; 4. Animals: Instincts 5. Houses: security: together or falling apart; 6. Falling: out of control, unsupported; 7. Chased: Identity resolution; 8. Water: Emotions: Calm or turbulent; 9. Sex: Trust or no trust; 10. Spider: Web (world) complexity; 11. Teeth: Losing face; 12: Transportation vehicle: movement (rushed or stagnant)

E

Electromagnetic Field, EMF
Normal EMF is what is created by nature or our bodies. Unnatural EMF is created by manmade machines or technology.

Electrical Trauma and Exposure, ETE
Electrocution or exposure to high voltage sources

Emotion: An affective state of consciousness in which joy, sorrow, fear, hate or the like is experienced. Emotion is a state of feeling and a feeling is the sensate experience of the emotion (Macquarie Concise Dictionary)

Emotion Energy: "negative" emotion has the potential to be "positive". It's only energy. We don't judge each end of the magnet as good or bad; similarly it's counterproductive to judge an emotion as good or bad. Emotion energy manifests as a vibration frequency.

Emotion Vibration language: a continuous pattern of vibration frequencies can be recorded erased (cleared), tuned, echoed, and stored in the cellular matrix. Cells continually echo stored frequencies.

Emotional balancing: Positive Affirmations**

Entities: There is an EMF association with the supernatural, otherwise, Sam and Dean Winchester[40] would not be using Gauss meters. One participant claimed that fear was so real to her that it was a shapeless being that she could feel near her. During the EVOX, I told her to try speaking to fear to leave and there was a release. In Case Study 9, there was a discharge release that coincidentally caused a brown-out in the area of and including our office. It is the Christian belief that entities cannot possess our soul unless invited but they can attach. What if they electrically attach to our EMF? What if the EVOX helps dislodge them?

EVOX: The EVOX protocols are non-drug, non-talk and non-invasive techniques based on the premise that they will reduce harmful, negative emotions on an energetic level. They use electronic frequencies customized to an individual's emotional state voice map. The change in emotional state should change the individual's perception of their emotional issue.

1. Testimonials - Promotional, http://www.youtube.com/watch?v=okWU6RulqBc
2. Testimonials – insight, compassion, instincts, lighter, potential, performance. Defines voice mapping, http://www.youtube.com/watch?v=VfeHXhRbNKA
3. Fear of water, http://www.youtube.com/watch?v=OsjbHKahSow
4. Explains clearing cellular memory in connective tissue using biofeedback http://www.youtube.com/watch?v=QJ5r9gfWWxg
5. Water holds memory. Mental blocks, http://www.youtube.com/watch?v=vriQFoqMVqU
6. Testimonial – Empowered, emotional healing, http://www.youtube.com/watch?v=fZfAumY9or0
7. Testimonial – Gratitude, http://www.youtube.com/watch?v=hkvzB_Jf1ww

F

Farmer's Almanac: (see Maunder's[41] work on astronomy in the bible)

---

[40] Characters in the series, "Supernatural" on CW TV.

Using of astronomy for agriculture.

Fear: emotion is one of the lowest vibrational frequencies and one of the highest propensities to result in a physiological condition.

Feelings: describes the sensate experience of the emotion. I feel sad, angry, joyful, fearful, and so on.

Fractals: Self similar patterns to represent geometric shapes in nature.

Freedom Perspective*: Awakening

Furnace Faith Perspective*: Mind over Matter, Tony Robbins's Walk of Fire.

G

Galvanic skin response (GSR): Skin stress response reflective of electrical meridians

Generational Iniquity: Transgenerational Effect
Renounce ancestral curses pasted down in families. Exodus 34:7, "Keeping mercy for thousands, forgiving iniquity and transgression and sin, and that will by no means clear the guilty; visiting (punishing) the iniquity of the fathers upon the children, and upon the children's children, unto the third and to the fourth generation." Lamentations 5:7, "Our fathers have sinned, and are not; and we have borne (been punished for) their iniquities."

Gluon: Universal Glue
Quarks and gluons are virtual particles of light and sound that are at the origin of all matter (2010 Nobel Prize for physics).

H

Happy: When our state of mind is pleasant most of the time (Maxwell Maltz).

Healing: Spontaneous or miraculous recovery
If the reality is that we create our own misfortunes by believing a lie, then, we can stop it! We can create happiness, wealth and healing by believing the truth. "But he *was* wounded for our transgressions; *he was* bruised for our iniquities: the chastisement of our peace *was* upon him;

---

[41] http://www.gutenberg.org/files/28536/28536-h/28536-h.htm

and with his stripes we are healed." Isaiah 53:5 The instruction I have received from Dan Bennett at Gateway Church is that if you do not recognize and acknowledge that salvation is a package deal there are consequences. You received the mind of Christ, the Holy Spirit and the Healing of the Body. So, open your mind's eye and see it. Open the eyes of your heart, and see it. See His report and not the world's report. "Therefore, whoever eats the bread or drinks from the cup in an unworthy manner will be held responsible for the Lord's body and blood". 1 Corinthians 11:27

Higgs Boson: "God particle," is believed to be the particle which gives mass to matter. The "God particle" nickname grew out of the long, drawn-out struggles of physicists to find this elusive piece of the cosmic puzzle.

Homeopathy: High dilutions of a substance until only the energy field remains.

Homeopathic[42] miasm: energy field representation of a genetic predisposition to a specific symptom or behavior pattern handed down from ancestors. TGR is to interrupt the transference of this field or break energy patterns that hold a current posture.

I

Information Field: The universal knowledge of all things: creation, structure, function plan and purpose of each atom to Adam (past, present and future).

Intention: Motive behind a thought.

J

Jealousy is intolerance to a perceived rivalry or advantage.

K

Kinesiology: Muscle testing based on the body's energy meridians.

Kingdom Self: Spirit being of God's light.

L

---

[42] http://www.youtube.com/watch?v=ee__R_ITz8w

Law of Attraction: (Abundance Perspective*) Positive thoughts attract positive experiences.

M

Matter: Purposed into physical reality from the wave nature of the quantum field. Everything in our universe is part of and is comprised of the quantum field. Matter itself is made of waves. All matter in the universe is interconnected as and by quantum waves which have no boundary.

Medium: One who channels or a psychic.

Mind over Matter: (Furnace Faith Perspective) Focus and concentration can override a crisis situation.

N

Near Death Experiences, NDE: When one's consciousness leaves a body that has no vital signs.

Nirvana: Heaven

Noetic: Science of Consciousness, i.e. Institute of Noetic Science (IONS).

Non-local: Phenomenon not occurring at the originating location or not in the physical world.

O

Organ Transplantation Psychiatry (OTP): Originating in the US, a new branch of psychiatry has developed in order to deal with personality changes due to organ transplant.

Out of Body Experiences, OBE: Consciousness leaving a living body

P

Parable Symbolism
1. Scorpions: demons; 2. Attacking birds: demons; 3. Thorns: demons 4. Mountain: consciousness; 5. Kingdom: presence of God; 6. Seed: intention; 7. Vineyard: world; 8. Master or Father: God; 9. Fruit: Lives,

works; 10. Branches: Groups of people; 11. Fire: judgment; 12. Servant: The Lord's prophet.

Power to move things with thought Perspective*: Telekinesis

Prayer: Spirit communication, Channeling: Practice of communicating with God. Prayer accesses the channel to God. It would be nice if we could say or know that the EVOX can turn up the volume on hearing the answers to our prayers or in the delivery. "Call to me and I will show you things you didn't know before." Jeremiah 33:3

Psychic: One who has the ability to access the information field or Akashi Record.

Q

Quark: Smallest known particle in the universe. Has an unusual characteristic of having a fractional electric charge, unlike the proton and electron, which have integer charges of +1 and -1 respectively. Has a charge called color charge. A quark is basically a wave very close to a sound wave.

Quantum field: A subset of the zero point field. The quantum field occurs as a result of the interaction of the electromagnetic waves of the zero point field and the subatomic particles of the quantum field. The interaction results in scalar waves.

R

Receiving Information Perspective: Download

Reframing perception: enlarging the view frame around our perceived reality to get the whole picture. Change your perception, change your reality.

Releasing Pattern: This is the indicator that the percentages noted on each voice map going in a counterclockwise direction had increase sufficiently for a beneficial result. In terms of quantum energy: the perception focus was energetically shifted toward an ideal healing field.

S

Scalar Waves: Waves that do not have direction or spin but in reality are interference patterns that are transformed via a holographic fournier transformation into material reality. This transformation is conducted by consciousness.

Sorcery: Pharmacopoeia

Skin Conductance Response SCR: These responses are utilized as part of the polygraph or lie detector.

Soniceuticals: Vibrational nutrition for your emotional body.

Subconscious perception: a judgment (subconscious agreement about) of a person, thing or relationship.

Symbols: 'A picture paints a thousand words.' That's the reason why we dream and parables are in symbols. You can say a whole lot more with an image than you can with a sentence.

T

Traumas: An occurrence recorded as physical or emotional low frequency vibration in connective tissue memory patterns. Instances documented as being passed on in organ transplant.

Transgenerational Reframing (TGR)[43]: Addresses Generational Iniquity. It is a Zyto Evox technique for Global Perspectives to reframe ancestral inertia.

Transcend: To rise above human understanding.

U

Universal Glue: Gluon

V

Visualization: (Think on things perspective) See using your mind's eye.

W

Wall Collapsing Perspective: Cymatic precision drop of a structure.

---

[43] http://www.youtube.com/watch?v=BdeLFb-EK5Y

Word of God Perspective: Inspired Living Document, Extrasensory Perception (ESP)

Y

Yahweh Breath: Fiat, something from nothing.

Yoga: (Temple worship perspective) It is a physical, mental, and spiritual practice of exercise, relaxation and meditation that originated in India.

Z

Zen: (Kingdom Living Perspective) Meditative state to attain enlightenment.

Zero-point energy: The vibrational energy retained by molecules even at a temperature of absolute zero.

Zyto: Bio-communication instrument.
1. Defines stress, homeostasis, residual stressors, stressor support, Galvanic Skin Response
http://www.youtube.com/watch?v=bCtLTVFlhz4
2. Defines biological preference, bio communication
http://www.youtube.com/watch?v=bh9tx14JthM

*See *Quantum Conscience* manual for references and details.

www.ingramcontent.com/pod-product-compliance
Lightning Source LLC
Chambersburg PA
CBHW070133290526
45789CB00005B/2227